Your Healing Diet

To order additional copies, please contact us.
BookSurge, LLC
www.booksurge.com
1-866-308-6235
orders@booksurge.com

Your Healing Diet
A Quick Guide to Reversing Psoriasis and
Chronic Diseases with Healing Foods

Deirdre Earls, RD, LD

2005

Your Healing Diet

Table of Contents

This is dedicated to Pop because I promised him that someday I'd write a book.

Introduction

"It would be possible to describe everything scientifically, but it would make no sense; it would be without meaning, as if you described a Beethoven symphony as a variation of wave pressure."—Albert Einstein

This guidebook is written to inspire you to experience the incredible healing power of food in the midst of very busy lifestyles. I invested hundreds of hours learning the shortcuts on how to research, shop, travel, cook and dine differently in order food to experience natural healing through food. To save you time and speed the benefits to you, I have distilled reams of information into this user-friendly, conversational guide.

Personal desperation initiated this journey. For over 25 years I struggled with severe psoriasis. Despite 15 years as a Registered Dietitian and 30 years of appointments with physicians around the world, I hadn't heard how food could create and reverse my skin condition.

In June 2002 my condition worsened and the skin on

my hands no longer allowed me to pick up a glass of water or open a jar. Expensive, chemotherapeutic drugs with horrible side effects had been recommended. In desperation I searched online and was introduced to a dietary approach that enables the body to heal itself. It was easy to understand why the diet supports natural healing. With nothing to lose but a disease and unwanted weight, I committed myself to this way of eating for 6 months. By December 2002 my hands had cleared almost completely, I lost 20 pounds and spent no money on prescription medications.

There are many healing diets including Macrobiotics, Raw Foods, Alkalizing, Anti-inflammatory, Cancer Prevention, Heart Disease Prevention and Anti-Aging Diets. These diets are associated with healing dozens of degenerative and autoimmune diseases. Like all of them, my approach to natural healing emphasizes whole grains, vegetables, legumes, fruits, nuts and seeds. Professional and personal experience taught me that healing diets are often ignored because it is difficult to practice them in the midst of busy lifestyles.

Although I respect the potential value of strict adherence to a healing diet, this book is written for those who have limited time to practice it completely. This guidebook is a 'fast food' version of sorts, meaning that the information is adapted to fit a busy lifestyle while still helping the body to achieve levels of natural healing. I have never been 100% compliant, and I occasionally eat foods that are strongly discouraged. But to my surprise, my less than perfect practice achieves remarkable healing. I wrote this book to help others experience the incredible healing power of food in a way that doesn't require seismic shifts in every dimension of life.

This book is written as a brief guide. It is not a medical study. Views presented herein on the genesis of disease, how food can reverse disease, and the diet suggestions themselves are merely my interpretations of research and how natural healing happened for me. I make no claim this information is scientifically proven nor that this is a guaranteed cure. My intent is simply to broaden your options for natural healing because 30 years of personal and professional experience showed me that this information isn't promoted in dietetics or western medicine. The choice is yours to decide if you will give food a chance to be your medicine.

Chapter One
Taking Control of Your Own Health

"Liberty means responsibility. That is why most men dread it." George Bernard Shaw

With all the anxieties of any newly minted adolescent, I was 13 and walking into my first day at Central Junior High School. One thing made me particularly self-conscious that day. Sometime over the preceding summer, severe psoriasis had erupted all over my body. Walking into a new school with hundreds of new faces, I knew I couldn't hide this reality. Quiet support from family and friends helped me to accept this problem and insist that it not rule my life.

25 years with psoriasis passed. Those years included 2 months in the hospital and thousands of dollars in drugs and doctors around the world. Some treatments would clear my skin for a couple of months, but quick relapses yielded a worsened condition. Powerful, expensive drugs emerged offering better results...and terrible side effects.

During this time, I graduated with honors in Scientific Nutrition from Texas A&M University. After completing a dietetic internship at The Indiana University Medical Center, I practiced as a Registered Dietitian for almost 15 years. Throughout this 20 year phase of my career, I heard nothing of what diet could do for my skin.

The turning point came in June of 2002. All of a sudden I couldn't unscrew jars or pick up a glass of water. Knuckles started to look arthritic and simply turning a steering wheel opened cracks in my hands. I was desperate and knew that a trip to the doctor would yield a prescription for methotrexate, a chemotherapy used to treat breast cancer. Like other prescription medication options for psoriasis, it offers brief relief, long-term side effects, and costly medical bills.

Anxious to be free of strong prescription medications, I went online and started searching for anything related to psoriasis. To my surprise, 'diet' started appearing. Several sources taught me that psoriasis happens when one eats foods to which they have an allergy or sensitivity. Perhaps in conjunction with an acid-forming diet and proliferation of damaging intestinal microbes, the allergic response renders a "leaky gut". Subsequent toxic seepage leads to a series of autoimmune responses, the consequences of which can be psoriasis or many other degenerative diseases like arthritis, heart disease, diabetes, and cancer.

With nothing to lose, I committed myself to natural healing with food. At first I was amazed at how much better I felt. Then I was struck at how quickly friends told me that my entire persona was changing. I embarked upon hundreds of hours in research and cooking classes that taught me how to use food to heal. The more I practiced a healing diet, the faster my skin healed. Sometimes the new demands and requisite patience were overwhelming, but encouragements to persevere kept me focused.

Symptoms typically worsen before they improve when one pursues natural healing. This happened to me and it took 5 months before my symptoms began to visibly improve. After six months, my hands and allergies had healed almost completely, I had lost 20 pounds of unwanted weight, and I had spent no money on prescription medications or physician appointments.

I have enormous gratitude for finding a solution that relieved my skin with no negative side effects, slashed food and medical costs, helped me lose over 20 pounds, and set me free from dependency on doctors and drugs. Knowing that this dietary solution isn't regularly promoted in dietetics or Western Medicine, I was inextricably drawn to share this diet and my knowledge in diet education to help others achieve the same benefits.

Personal experience and years of nutrition education taught me that even in desperate situations, dietary habits can be very difficult to change. My mission is to help you take control of your health via a diet that promotes natural healing and fits your busy lifestyle, thereby enhancing compliance and probability for long-term success.

Chapter Two
The Big Experiment

"Take the first step in faith. You don't have to see the whole staircase, just take the first step." Martin Luther King, Jr.

After committing to a six month experiment to see how diet might affect my psoriasis, I embarked upon hundreds of research hours. The online information ranged from international medical sites to home remedies to books. Across multitudes of sources, I looked for common threads of success. These common threads included the importance of avoiding animal products (beef, chicken and dairy), refined sugars, refined flours, processed foods, alcohol, fatty foods, hydrogenated fats and spicy foods. There also seemed to be a frequent connection between gluten intolerance and autoimmune problems like psoriasis. Meat, wine, cheese and jalapenos were dietary staples and parting with them was not easy. But the more I studied, the more I knew I had nothing to lose ... except a disease, unwanted weight and destructive habits, unwanted weight and destructive habits. Additionally, it was obvious that this diet would protect me from obesity, heart disease, diabetes and cancer.

My first step towards practicing natural healing came after reading a book by an American chiropractor, Dr. John Pagano. In approximately 300 pages of his book, "Healing Psoriasis; The Natural Alternative", his recommendations include diet, enemas and colonics, spinal adjustments, various ointments and specific baths. Although I deeply appreciate the value of his work, I wasn't comfortable with many of his recommendations and subsequently focused solely on those which I knew to contribute no harm, namely the diet, an optimistic outlook and regular outdoor activity.

Within a week of diet change, I had a very deep and rare sense of knowing that I was doing the right thing. I could feel my whole body breathing a sigh of relief. Soon friends were commenting on my new "glow" and the positive change in my persona. I explained Dr. Pagano's diet and many likened it to other healing diets. Across much research I found that all the healing diets encourage a daily preponderance of organic vegetables and fruits. Most of the healing diets also appeared to take a severe stance towards compliance with their diet. Years of work as a hospital dietitian taught me the wastefulness of simply lecturing on radical diet change. Very few people adhere to strict diets for long periods of time. It is much more useful and effective to educate on how to integrate good habits into an individual's unique lifestyle. This is especially true when attempting to achieve natural healing with food. The process is slow and invariably requires patience. I constantly remind my clients, "Two steps forward, one step back."

I continued researching all types of healing diets. Unlike Dr. Pagano's diet, many other healing diets encourage exclusion of dairy, meat and chicken while including small amounts of fish. I decided to eliminate all animal products except fish as part of my experiment. To the extent that I eliminated animal products and incorporated more alkalizing plants into my diet, my skin and allergies cleared much more quickly than they did while I practiced Dr. Pagano's diet. I've never turned back.

Importantly, I learned that a healing diet built upon whole grains and fresh produce is a way of eating that enhances health, prevents disease and promotes natural healing <u>for everyone</u>, not just for those with psoriasis.

Chapter Three
How Food can Create and Reverse Disease.... Slowly

"Success seems to be connected with action. Successful men keep moving. They make mistakes, but they don't quit." Conrad Hilton

In the first chapter I introduced a possible genesis of many diseases, namely that poor elimination and ingestion of certain foods and toxins can damage the lining of the intestines and create a leaky gut. In conjunction with an acid-forming diet and proliferation of damaging bacteria and parasites, toxins subsequently leak into the bloodstream and ultimately create overload on our filtering organs. The liver filters blood and the kidneys filter water. As the liver and kidneys are increasingly taxed with greater toxic volume, they start shuttling the extra toxins to other elimination organs like the skin and the lungs. Hence, our body alerts us to early stages of illness via discharge of these extra toxins at these areas. This is when we develop colds, sinus congestion, coughing, sneezing, excessive sweating and minor skin irritations. Unresolved seepage of pollutants from the intestines leads to further toxic build up in the body. Acute problems become chronic problems of the skin, hair and nails, along with chronic colds and flu, and general fatigue. If the cause of the problem is not corrected, the body's elimination methods are increasingly taxed and the body begins to accumulate more damaging levels of toxins at deeper levels. This yields more serious problems in other discharge areas of the body like the joints, ears, tonsils, breasts, uterus, sinuses, gums, lungs. Rheumatoid arthritis, lupus, fibromyalgia, mononucleosis, shingles and other autoimmune disorders are likely to develop at this stage of accumulation. Further toxic accumulation demands that the body store toxins in ever deeper areas, ultimately producing degenerative alterations in vital organs. Most major diseases including cancers, cardiovascular disease, and diabetes arise at this point. Some view these diseases as the body's natural means of isolating pollutants in tumors and organs instead of allowing toxins to systemically overwhelm the bloodstream, yielding more immediate death. This uncanny ability of our body not only 'buys time' but also offers the opportunity to reflect on how our choices directly influence our condition and to change accordingly.

Now that you understand this theory on the progression of disease, it's important to understand how food can reverse disease. First, by eliminating the foods which weaken the intestinal lining and feed bad microbes, you stop contributing to intestinal damage and provide necessary relief for healing of that tissue. As you stop the intestinal damage, you'll also halt the leaking of toxins and thereby give the body's filtration and immune systems a well deserved break. As your choices no longer contribute to an overtaxed immune system, you'll allow it to regain its ability to discharge toxins instead to storing them. And by including healing foods into your diet, you'll be providing the necessary nutrition and environment to build healthy tissue and blood. This renders natural healing throughout the body.

One of the wonderful things about natural healing is being

able to view the sequential consequences of good decisions, and to experience how good choices perpetuate themselves with more positives. In other words, **to the extent that you demonstrate respect and gratitude for your body by making choices that nurture instead of damage it, you experience a long series of positive responses.** Almost immediately you feel better and recognize the sense that you're doing the right thing.

However, despite this simple logic for natural healing, adopting this way of eating was anything but easy. It was the most difficult thing I have ever done because I was so attached to my old eating habits. The good news is that this new way of eating ultimately becomes its own habit, and you start to crave how quality food makes you feel. You recognize the difference in your energy, moods and vitality. To the extent that you are compliant, you will feel the difference. And this feeling will act as a strong motivator to keep you compliant long before you see symptom improvement.

It is important to mention that when one decides to address the cause of disease, one decides to go inward and heal more completely from the inside out, versus healing only the symptoms from the outside in. This inward discipline and natural healing requires time. The natural healing process is almost always slower than that of prescription medications, so it requires patience, persistence and commitment. Natural healing is rarely an overnight phenomenon, so you shouldn't expect an immediate improvement in your symptoms. In general, the longer you've experienced symptoms, the greater the amount of toxic accumulation and the longer it takes to discharge that accumulation from the body.

In fact, symptoms regularly worsen before they improve. After diet change, the body's elimination systems have strengthened and gained greater ability to discharge. The extra discharge causes symptoms to temporarily worsen. When symptoms worsen it is imperative to persevere. Continue visualizing the desired result and don't quit. These phases of healing are the most difficult. It is discouraging to radically change one's diet and then experience worsening symptoms. However, when you experience this, know that you are on the right track. During this phase of my healing, my condition was more painful and itched more than I had ever experienced. Four months into diet change, night itching was so terrible that I often wanted to jump out of my skin and I understood how unresolved itch could drive someone insane. My ankles were so tight and hot that I had to sleep with my feet off the edge of the bed. The heat and the itching regularly woke me up in the middle of the night. This was undoubtedly the most challenging phase of my healing. I had given up so many beloved foods and the social experiences that went along with them, only to see my condition worsening. To stay focused, I read and reread pages in books on natural healing that explained that this type of flare up was an indication that I was healing and releasing more discharge from within. I persisted and after six weeks my healing took a huge turn for the better. Symptoms began to vanish and I have remained in remission for years.

Once your symptoms clear and you experience the incredible healing power of food, you'll be aware of a multitude of benefits:

1)   The emotional relief that comes from having control over your health and symptoms. This might be the first time you've experienced any control over your symptoms and the disease.

2)   You'll be less dependent upon prescription medications and liberated from a very complicated medical system.

3)   You'll have more money in your pocket. Your food costs will probably decrease when you stop buying animal products and alcohol. Fewer prescription

medications and fewer trips to the doctor inevitably mean more money in your pocket, too.

4) If you have other health problems, they might improve, too. For instance, I had chronic allergy and sinus problems before changing my diet. A lifetime of allergy problems are now virtually gone.

5) I always emphasize alleviating the cause of disease over weight loss. But you can expect to lose weight and experience the positive health and self-image benefits of weight loss.

But to achieve natural healing with food, I must stress the combined importance of a deliberate diet, patience and persistence. All three are equally critical for success.

Chapter Four
Healing Principles—Diet, Positive Outlook, Outdoor Activity

"In essence, holistic healing is properly setting in motion the forces of nature within the individual that will help the body to heal itself." Dr. John O.A. Pagano, Chiropractic Physician
"The goal of macrobiotics is freedom—the ability to create and realize our dream in life..." Michio Kushi

Many healing diets offer a multipronged approach to true health. They all iterate the importance of being in harmony within your own body and within the larger forces of nature. In addition to diet they emphasize the significance of a positive outlook, a grateful attitude and symbiotic interaction with nature. In theory they might say that according to each individual, no food is prohibited and no food alone will heal. However, my humble opinion is that they often reflect an extreme position towards a lifestyle which strictly excludes many foods and practices. Perhaps because of their demands across every dimension of life, I frequently heard reports of binging and abandoning these diets.

My intent is to help you bridge the distance between these extremes and what you can realistically accomplish. You should feel good about your achievement—even when it's not perfect. After an initial six month period of cleansing, I encourage flexibility because flexibility is crucial for long-term compliance. And long-term compliance is necessary for natural healing because the process is inherently slow. My hunch is that this orientation will minimize binging and facilitate a more positive outlook, which in turn will enhance the chances of accepting this way of eating for the rest of your life. *For it's what we choose to eat on a daily basis over many years that is the key to preventing and reversing disease naturally with food.*

Chapter six details the dietary approach but the basics of how to eat for good health are neither trendy nor new. They're the same dietary recommendations that we've already heard a million times before, namely:

1)   Increase consumption of complex carbohydrates (especially whole grains and fresh vegetables and fresh fruits) and reduce consumption of refined sugars (white sugar, cane juices, high fructose corn syrups, etc);

2)   Decrease consumption of animal foods like meats, poultry, eggs and dairy;

3)   Reduce total fat consumption, especially of saturated fats which are found in animal products like meat, poultry, eggs and dairy;

4)   Eat from a wide variety of fresh foods to secure a balance of vitamins and minerals, thereby decreasing or eliminating the need for supplementation;

5) Eat more <u>high fiber, simple, fresh and organic foods</u> and less chemically processed foods.

Other Healing Principles:

Simplicity:
Throughout human history, religious and philosophical leaders have emphasized the value of simplicity. So goes the inherent value of simplicity in food and food that is as close as possible to its original, whole form. Whole food contains more energy than the same food which has been processed and devitalized. For instance, when the tombs of Egypt were reopened, brown rice kernels were found. When water was added to those brown rice kernels, they sprouted. Hence, 4000 years after the grains were harvested, the grain was still edible and it still held a vital life force that allowed it to sprout and provide more life. In contrast, what would the archeologists have found if brown rice flour had been left in the tomb instead of whole grain brown rice kernels? It's no surprise that simple, whole foods provide the most vibrant life force and we can give our bodies more life force by choosing to eat foods with more of it. The choices we make for food, friends, environment, and work either give our body the energy to heal itself or they drain us and make us unhealthy.

Chewing:
Chew your food 50 times or more until it becomes liquid in your mouth. Saliva contains the alkaline enzyme, amylase, which facilitates digestion. The more we chew, the more we release amylase. Chewing also stimulates movement and flow within the lymph nodes under the chin. Some macrobiotic teachers have said that chewing your food 50+ times can cut the healing time in half.

Moderation and Avoidance of Extremes:

Expect and be prepared for hunger. This will help you to avoid binging on lower quality foods. In other words, always keep quality foods at your fingertips. Eat when you're hungry but try to avoid eating 3 hours before sleeping in order to give your digestive system a break. Avoid overeating. The notion of balance relies on universal harmony and balance instead of extremes in foods, thought and environment. Do the diet imperfectly, without beating yourself up, so that you can do it longer. A sustained commitment is obligatory for most types of natural healing, so include one or two 'sacred' foods on a limited basis to make it easier to avoid binging and constant feelings of deprivation. For example, I continued drinking coffee every morning as a way to trick my brain and keep it from focusing on thoughts of deprivation from sugar, alcohol, chicken and dairy.

Food Preparation:
From the standpoint that you are what you eat, we absorb nutrition and vibration from our foods. High quality food is not only simple, whole and free of genetic modification, but it is also grown and prepared to accomplish more than convenience. When you cook, do so with healthful, loving energy and thoughts. In contrast, modern food is highly refined and processed to maximize profit. Convenience foods are not only laden with artificial ingredients, but they also enable us to speed through meals and life. In the kitchen, instead of the consistent heat from a gas flame, microwave ovens and electrical devices create a chaotic vibration that enters our food and us. Returning to a simpler, less stressful way of eating that respects the life-giving quality of food is essential to recovering and maintaining good health and high spirits.

Seven Elements of Health:
Seven indicators of true health are endless energy, strong

appetite, deep sleep, strong memory, peaceful mind, being joyful and alert, and endless appreciation.

Positive Outlook:

Adopting this diet was the most difficult thing I have ever done. Patience, persistence and right thinking are critical to sustain successful diet change. It's no surprise that approaching diet change in a relaxed, confident way will make it easier to accept and practice. This lifestyle change may be one of the most demanding changes of your life because food serves to provide not only nutrition, but comfort, pleasure and social context. To radically alter how one eats requires not only a change in the food but also a change in attitude that respects your body and prioritizes a commitment to health over instantaneous gratification.

Progress is rarely linear so I constantly remind my clients, "Two steps forward, one step back." To stay focused despite inevitable setbacks and occasional binges, it's important to habitually give yourself affirmative messages. When I craved wine, sweets, and spicy foods, I'd repeat positive messages like, "I choose to eat for health. Every day I'm getting better and the diet is easy to follow." Instead of beating yourself up for temporary binges, focus on the positives and regularly congratulate yourself on your examples of self-discipline.

Good, Better, Best:

This principle represents the decision process we have in food selection. I love this principle because it refrains from labeling 'bad' decisions and instead focuses on positives and leaves no associated guilt. Depending upon our commitment level at the moment we choose to eat, we make 'good, better or best' choices.

Chapter Five
The Acid/Alkaline Balance and Why a Healing Diet Works

"I've never seen a disease that did not have a mineral deficiency as its root cause." Linus Pauling
"The human body functions best when our blood is slightly alkaline. We make acid as a natural by-product of metabolism, but we make no alkaline. We must therefore get alkalinizing minerals from our diets."—<u>Cancer Battle Plan Sourcebook</u>, Dr. Dave Frahm, 2000, Penguin Putnam Inc., New York, page 147.
"Even a mild stressor can cause a partial or total acid-forming reaction," <u>Alkalize or Die</u>, Dr. Theodore A. Baroody, Jr., 1993, Eclectic Press, Waynesville, NC 28786, page 157.

We've talked about how removing irritating foods and pollutants from the diet will allow intestines to heal and stop more toxins from seeping into the bloodstream. The consumption of certain foods and a positive outlook provide the necessary fiber, nutrition and environment to allow the body to heal itself and ward off future disease. If toxins continue to be ingested, intestines continue to leak these poisons into the bloodstream creating hyperacidity and a potentially damaging pH in your body. Mindful elimination, consumption and outlook are critical in helping the body to establish proper alkalinity and the proper environment to heal itself.

According to the theory of evolution, we evolved from the sea. Therefore our bodies, like an ancient ocean, must remain alkaline. Our life depends upon the constant and highly sensitive maintenance of a blood pH of ~ 7.4.

With pH effects in mind, a balanced healthy lifestyle supports proper alkalinity via consciousness in diet, thought and activity. A healing diet is based around mineral rich plant foods that promote alkalinity. A positive outlook creates positive emotions and the ability to visualize the desired result. Habitually negative, damaging thoughts influence our internal biochemistry and produce acidic toxins. Activity, especially walking in nature, eases the mind and stimulates circulatory, respiratory and lymphatic systems. Increased exhalation with laughter and exercise rids our bodies of excess carbon dioxide, which is mildly acidic. **Hence, the combination of diet, thought and exercise is vital to creating the necessary alkaline internal environment for natural healing.**

First, a healing diet strongly emphasizes mineral rich foods that support proper alkalinity in the body. The majority of one's food intake should consist of alkaline-forming foods, namely organic vegetables and fruits. Chapter Six provides great detail on these alkaline- forming foods, how to find them, and how to integrate them into your lifestyle. Most vegetables, fruits, herbs and sprouts are alkaline-forming, as are some whole grains. By calling them "alkaline-forming", this means that they render an alkaline ash. By ash, I mean that the remains of digestion are an ash, just like the remains of a burned log on a fire are an ash. That ash has an acidic or an alkaline pH. Heavier, fattier foods like meat, dairy, fish, eggs, processed foods, grains, refined sugars and refined flours yield an acidic ash. A plant based diet of mineral rich foods, along with a positive outlook and regular physical activity will support alkalinity, a strong immune system and optimal health. A diet that's high in animal proteins and saturated fats, processed foods, refined flour and refined sugars, combined with destructive emotions and inactivity, render a hyper acidic, disease-prone condition. In general, alkalinity is strongly preferred, but inclusion of some acid-forming foods in the diet is essential for complete nutrition. When you are trying to recover naturally from disease, it is good to have a diet that is ~80% alkaline-forming and ~20% acid-forming. This is challenging but to the extent that the vast majority of your diet is built around whole grains, vegetables and fruits, you will alkalize your system. This will enhance the ability of your immune system to rid your body of toxins and create natural healing. After symptoms are resolved, you still want a majority of your intake to be alkaline-forming. A general guideline for maintaining optimal health is ~60% alkaline-forming and ~40% acid-forming.

On a separate but important note, when one's diet is acid-forming, the body inevitably has to deplete minerals from other sources to neutralize the acid. Because bones represent the largest and most readily available storage of alkalizing minerals, calcium is depleted from them until the blood and body tissues reach their proper pH. Calorie for calorie, most dark, leafy green vegetables contain not only more calcium than milk, but they also have a much better calcium to phosphorous ratio for increased bioavailability. Additionally, the saturated fat and high protein content in dairy contributes directly to acidity. Despite what we hear from the National Dairy Council, societies that regularly drink milk suffer widely from osteoporosis, whereas those with dairy-free or vegetarian diets do not.

Chapter Six
Healing Diet Basics

"Man must cease attributing his problems to his environment, and learn again to exercise his will— his personal responsibility." Albert Einstein

DIET BASICS

- Focus on organic whole grains, fresh vegetables (minus the nightshades for those with allergies, skin problems, arthritis) and fresh fruits. When in doubt, eat a plant.

- Although I achieved significant healing while buying non-organic produce, subsequent research convinced me of the value of avoiding their genetic modifications, herbicides and pesticides. Now I buy and eat organic produce whenever possible.

- Diseases like psoriasis, asthma, allergies, skin problems and arthritis are characterized by inflammation. If your condition involves inflammation, avoid the Nightshades and Citrus fruits. Nightshades include tomatoes, white potatoes, tobacco, eggplant, and any variety of peppers including bell, jalapeno, serrano, poblano, habanero, etc. Black pepper is not a nightshade. Nightshades are to be avoided because they contain solanine. Solanine contributes to inflammatory responses, especially in the joints. Citrus fruits include oranges, grapefruits, pineapple, lemons and lime. However, even for those with inflammation, it is good to squeeze small amounts of fresh lemon juice onto food or into water for an alkalizing effect.

- Avoid shellfish and filter-feeding fish (like shrimp, lobster, scallops, oysters, clams) as they feed of the sewage that floats down to them. Consumption of freely swimming fish should be limited to eight ounces per week.

- Excluding freely swimming fish, avoid all animal products including beef, pork, chicken, fowl, dairy and eggs. The saturated fat, antibiotics, hormones and higher protein content along with the pesticides in grains used to feed animals, are not conducive to natural healing. If craved, try to limit yourself to 4 oz per week of red meat, 8 oz per week of white chicken or fowl, 2 eggs per week, 8 oz. low- or nonfat yogurt, and 2 oz of low fat or nonfat cheese.

- The simpler the food the better. Once a food is no longer in its whole state, it has to be processed in some way to keep it from deteriorating. Fresh is always best, and frozen is the next best option. Canned, dried and fried foods should be rarely eaten.

- Drink filtered, distilled or spring water instead of chlorinated tap water. The chlorine in tap water kills the good bacteria in our gut. Additionally, tap water frequently contains toxic residues and metals.

- Avoid all alcohol including wine, beer and liquor.

- Avoid products made with refined white sugars, high fructose corn syrup and any type of cane juice.

- Check with your physician before embarking upon significant diet change.

- If you determine you are allergic to a food, avoid it even if it is on this list. Many people have allergies to wheat (gluten intolerance), corn, soy and dairy. Those with gluten intolerance should avoid wheat, barley, oats, rye, spelt and kamut. In general, wheat is the biggest culprit so I try to avoid it entirely. I occasionally eat spelt and oats.

- In general food offers superior nutrition when compared to supplements. But for those who can not or will not practice a healing diet, supplements might be recommended. The only supplement that I regularly take is Cod Liver Oil.

- READ INGREDIENT LABELS LIKE A HAWK! Tricky marketing exists in many areas of 'healthy' food products. The simpler and the shorter the ingredient labels, the better. Choose products made of recognizable foods instead of synthetic laboratory ingredients with unfamiliar names.

- Don't let yourself get hungry. When I'm really hungry and don't have quality food at my fingertips, I invariably get frustrated and eat whatever is available. Pack healthy snacks in your refrigerator, car, purse and office to ensure you always have quality food at your fingertips. Almond butter, raisins, Odwalla bars, LaraBars, fiber-rich juices (like Odwalla Superfood or Naked Juices or Amazake) and brown rice cakes are great snacks which can travel almost anywhere.

Rough dietary guidelines include ~ 40% of daily calories in whole grains; ~20% in vegetables; ~15% in seeds or nuts or beans or fish; ~15% in fruit; ~5-10% in oils; ~5% in vegetable soups and sea vegetables.

Whole Grains:

Whole grains comprise ~40% of daily food intake. Except in cases of gluten intolerance, any whole grains are allowed and brown rice acts as the daily whole grain staple. Whole grain varieties include brown rice, corn, millet, amaranth, kamut, teff, spelt, oatmeal, buckwheat, kasha, bulgar, quinoa, triticale, wheat, barley, rye.

From a nutritional and energetic standpoint, eating whole grains is best and less processing is always better. Each step of processing or refining a food will devitalize it and compromise its nutrition. Hence, brown rice is superior to brown rice flour, steel cut oats are superior to oatmeal flakes, and fresh corn is superior to corn meal. White flour and other highly refined and polished grains are always avoided. Whole grain flours are acceptable on an occasional basis in bagels, breads, muffins, cereals. Gluten intolerance from wheat products is an issue in several auto-immune diseases like psoriasis. Hence, I avoid all wheat products and now base my diet around brown rice and corn.

Vegetables:

About 20% of the daily food should include fresh vegetables which can be prepared in any number of ways, but frying should be avoided. Fresh vegetables are the highest in energy, minerals and nutrients. Opinions differ and research hasn't concluded whether it's better to eat raw versus lightly cooked vegetables, but overcooking vegetables will definitely compromise the nutrition they can deliver to you. I most often eat raw vegetables.

All vegetables are allowed <u>except</u> the nightshades in cases of inflammatory conditions like psoriasis and arthritis. (The nightshades include tomatoes, all types of peppers, white potatoes, eggplant and tobacco.) Dark, leafy green vegetables are to be eaten as often as possible as they are very alkalizing. These dark, leafy vegetables include bok choy, arugula, kale, turnip greens, mustard greens, collard greens, watercress, herbs like basil and parsley and cilantro, leeks, spinach, lettuce varieties, Chinese cabbage, carrot tops, daikon tops, beet tops, Swiss chard, scallions, dandelion greens, broccoli rabe, pak choy and Chinese gai lan. Other allowable vegetables include sweet potatoes, yams, string and wax beans, endive, escarole, red and green cabbage, mushrooms, artichoke varieties, carrots, onions, garlic, shallots, sugar snap peas, broccoli, cauliflower, Brussels sprouts, asparagus, parsnips, turnips, corn, all squashes, zucchini, beets, olives, celery, fennel, cucumber, garlic, avocado, artichokes. Vegetable juicing provides good nutrition but because the fiber and some minerals are removed, I prefer to eat vegetables whole instead of juiced.

Seeds, Nuts, Beans and Fish:

For protein sources, about 15% of daily food includes seeds, nuts and beans of any variety and fish. Almonds are the only nuts that are alkalizing and hence they are encouraged more than the other nuts. Tofu, tempeh, seitan and natto, all of which are soybean products, may be taken daily. Grilled, baked, sautéed, steamed or poached fish is recommended twice weekly. Fresh white water varieties are preferred. More highly recommended fish include cod, albacore, bass, mahi mahi, flounder, fluke, grouper, haddock, halibut, perch, red snapper, salmon, sardines, scrod, sole-sturgeon, swordfish, trout, and whitefish. However, research is indicating that swordfish and salmon can be high in toxic mercury. Therefore, I avoid swordfish and eat light chunk tuna or wild salmon at a maximum of eight ounces per week. In the shopping section I have provided ordering information on a tuna that is low in mercury.

Fruit:

About 15% of daily intake comes from fruits, and whole fruit is always preferable to juices because whole fruit provides beneficial fiber and minerals. Nevertheless, if you drink juice, make sure that it's fresh and includes no refined sugars or cane juice.

All fruits are allowed. Fruits that are frozen and packed in water or fruit juice are occasionally permitted but fresh fruits are always best. Strawberries and Citrus Fruits (oranges, orange juice, grapefruits, pineapple, lemon and limes) are often discouraged for arthritis, psoriasis and psoriatic arthritis. Freshly squeezed lemon or lime can be added to drinking water or used in dressings for a cleansing and alkalizing effect.

Oils:

Oils comprise ~ 5—10% of daily caloric intake. Olive oil is the most frequently recommended oil. Canola, Safflower, Corn, Cottonseed, Soybean, sunflower, sesame and peanut oils are OK. Salad dressings are best with olive oil and fresh squeezed lemon juice or apple cider vinegar. Avoid heating oils, or rancid oils that are exposed to light and heat. If possible and the recipe allows, I cook without oil and add olive oil after a food is cooked. Macadamia nut and coconut oils are known for their ability to sustain nutrition integrity at higher temperatures.

Soups and Sea Vegetables:

Soups and sea vegetables comprise about 5% of food intake.

Vegetable soups can be made from any vegetables. It is ideal to season the soup with miso, but never add miso to boiling water because boiling water will kill the good bacteria in it. Vegetable soups, bean soups and grain soups are all recommended and allow for extra variety.

A small volume of sea vegetable is taken daily. Sea vegetables are frequently used in sushi, miso soup or when cooking rice. Nori, wakame, kombu, hijiki, arame, dulse, sea palm and Irish moss are included. These veggies are dense with minerals and therefore very alkalizing. Try to include at least a small portion of these in your daily diet. I've not developed a taste for them so I'm always looking for ways to hide their sea flavor. For instance, I cook brown rice with kombu, shake dulse granules from a condiment shaker onto salads and rice dishes, snack on brown rice cakes with seaweed, and dip nori sheets into hummus. Sea vegetables are essentially dark, leafy green vegetables which have derived their mineral density from the ocean floor and the salty sea water. They are alkalizing superfoods. Add them in any way possible to your daily diet.

Always Avoid:

Non-organic beef and non-organic chicken and their fats. Non-organic dairy and dairy milk fat. All white sugar, corn syrups and cane juices. All white flour. White rice. More than

1 glass of wine per week. Coffee. Nitrates and all processed meats like bologna and sausage and hot dogs. Tobacco. Shellfish like shrimp, lobster, oysters and scallops which are filter feeders that consume sewage from the sea floor. Junk food and processed foods like sodas. Trans-fatty acids and partially hydrogenated fats in packaged foods and fast foods. All fried foods. Sweets and pastries. Artificial sweeteners and colors. Sugary cereals. Spicy ingredients except tumeric.

Chapter Seven
At the Grocery Store

Shopping can be overwhelming when you revise your dietary choices to exclude dairy, chicken, red meat, wheat, sodas, alcohol, spicy foods, sweets, and refined flour products. This chapter provides lists of specific foods and their brands along with where you can find them. This list is by no means representative of the only things you should buy. Rather, the list provides general guidelines to help people anywhere understand how to make grocery store choices. The brands are not necessarily the best ones for this diet, they just happen to be the ones I purchase from specific grocery stores below. When I changed my diet, I got into a new 'routine' at the grocery store. Routines are helpful because they're fast and reflexive and don't require time to think through decisions. This list was developed to make it easier and faster for you to redo your routine at any grocery store.

General shopping suggestions include:

1) If particular foods are especially tempting because they're associated with your old habits or addictions, avoid them altogether. Don't even look at them.

2) Don't go to the grocery store hungry. Even if

you don't feel hungry before going to the store, eat something in advance of shopping to lessen impulsive temptations.

3) Buy some items that aren't exactly perfect to allow for occasional moments of feeling indulged rather than deprived.

4) Keep a few prized items on hand at all times to decrease your chances of binging. For example, in the past, I didn't allow myself the 'expense' of precut fresh fruit. Then I realized that by eliminating animal products and alcohol, I save plenty of money to buy precut fruits. Keeping some precut fruit in my refrigerator ensures that I always have something sweet and high quality at my fingertips for those times when I'm craving sweetness. I also buy bars like LaraBars and Nectar bars. Their ingredients are simple and they travel well. If I'm on road trips or stuck in traffic or at a party where there's nothing for me to eat, or nowhere near a grocery store, I'm very grateful to have LaraBars at my fingertips. Moments when it's impossible to quickly access quality food arise every day, so ensure that you're prepared with quality snacks. As my hunger rises, willpower falls. The key is to avoid real hunger. Other ways that I fulfill a sweet urge include making fruit smoothies and drinking packaged fruit smoothies like Sambazon Acai or Naked Juice's Green Machine. Although I still stumble and sometimes stumble badly, there are always better options for a sweet tooth than frozen dairy products, chocolate, candies and pastries.

Austin Shopping Lists

** **Indicates that I frequently buy this product at this particular location. It might not be available at other stores,**

or this designated store might provide the best price I've found for this product. In other words, ** means that I buy this product and when I buy it , I buy it at the designated store because this store offers the best price I've found or the product hasn't been located anyplace else in Austin.

At Costco:
**Martinelli's organic apple juice
**Odwalla's Superfood and B-Monster Juices
Walnuts, Almonds, Roasted Peanuts, Pine Nuts
**Cuisinart Blender/Food Processor
**Organic mixed spring greens for salads
**Frozen white fish filets (orange roughy, sea bass, cod)
Fresh Fish Fillets (tilapia, salmon, tuna, halibut)
**Frozen blueberries, frozen berries, Frozen Mango chunks
**Ruta Maya organic coffee
Portabella mushrooms
Pitted Kalamata Olives
Garden of Eatin's Organic Blue Tortilla Chips
Fresh Corn
Seedless Watermelon
**Fresh cut Fruit Tray with melons and pineapple
French Cut Green Beans, Green Asparagus, Sweet Corn on the Cob
Uncle Luke's 100% Pure Maple Syrup
**Cliff Bars
Cod Liver Oil Capsules
Cetaphil cleanser and moisturizer
Aveeno Skin Care products

At Whole Foods:
**Organic Burdock Root and Daikon Radish
**Nature's Path Instant Plain Hot Oatmeal in packets
**Nature's Path Organic fruit sweetened Corn flakes
**Lundberg Farms' Tamari and Seaweed Brown Rice Cakes
**LaraBars, Odwalla Bars

**Large Variety of Gluten-free and Whole Grain pastas
Vegenaise
**Miso Mayo (Vegetarian mayonnaise containing miso—
  Garlic & Dill, Original Flavor)
**Miso Soup in To Go packets
Freshly Ground Almond Butter
Sorrel Ridge 100% Fruit Spreads
**Fiordifrutta Organic 100% fruit spreads
**Amy's Frozen Organic Brown Rice Bowls and other Frozen
  Meals
**Organic Dolmas
**Emerald Valley Organic Hummus Varieties
**Rudi's Organic Whole Spelt Tortillas
**Food for Life's Sesame Spelt Bread with no yeast
**Wheat Free Raspberry Fig Bars
**Sardines in Olive Oil
**Tumeric
** Amazake organic rice shakes
**Date Coconut Rolls
** Sambazon's Organic Acai Energy Drinks
**Organic Cold Pressed Extra Virgin Olive Oil
**Brown Jasmine Rice
**Lundberg Farm Brown Rice varieties

At **Central Market at 38th street and Lamar:**
**Organic Brown Basmati Rice
**Arrowhead Mills Organic Multigrain, Amaranth, Spelt,
  Kamut Flake Cereals
**Arrowhead Mills Puffed Millet, Kamut, Corn, Brown Rice
  Cereals
**Spicy Dipping Sauce
Organic Sugar Snap Peas
**Rapini / Broccoli Raabe
**Pacific Brand Almond Milk
**Bulk Ground Almond Butter, Cashew Butter, Peanut
  Butter

100% fruit spreads
**Organic Lemons
**Rice Crackers with Tamari and Seaweed
**Bulk Basil Pesto
Organic Frozen Veggies: Corn, Peas, Mixes
**Lundberg Farm Organic Brown Rice Mixes
**Fresh Fish Fillets (Tilapia, Cod, Salmon, Halibut, Mahi Mahi, Orange Roughy)
**Santa Cruz's Unsweetened Organic Apple sauces

At HEB:

General Organic Produce: Organic Arugula, Celery, Carrots, Beets, Kale, Cabbage, Romaine, Scallions, Turnips, Leeks, Bananas, Grapes
Bob's Red Mill Steel Cut Oats
**Martin Brother's Tamari Vinaigrette and Thai Peanut Dressings
**Sass' Lemon Song and Sesame Garlic Dressings
**Oka's Miso Dressing
**Bulk Tamari Almonds, Dates, Chilean Raisins, Unsweetened Dehydrated Bananas
**Robert's American Gourmet Veggie Booty and Fruity Booty
**Barbara's Natural Choice Granola Bars (with no cane juice)
Whole and Pre-Cut Watermelon
**Naked Juice's 100% pureed fruit smoothies
**Pre-cut Chinese Veggie Mix of Bamboo sprouts, Bok Choy, Onion, Celery, Cabbage.
Other Produce: Lacinato Kale, Butternut and Acorn Squash, Zucchini, Summer Squash, Asparagus, Avocado, Ginger, Red and White Button Onions, Shallots, Garlic, Sweet Potatoes, Sugar Snap Peas,

At Phoenicia Bakery on Burnet Road:
**Sultan Raisins

**Dried Cherries
Bulk Olive Bar
**Hummus
**Yogurt with Dill and Onions
Dried Figs
**Tuna and White Beans Salad
**Fava bean salad
Dolmas

At Casa de Luz Grocery Store on Toomey Road:
**Tohum's Organic Tahini
**Tohum's Organic Mulberry Extract
**Large Green Vegetable Storage Bags
**Natural Brushes for scrubbing Veggies and Fruits
**FrigoVerre Italian Glass Storage Bowls with Lids
**South River Miso and handmade Misos
Sea Seasonings Sea Vegetable Condiments
Organic Nori Rolls
Eden's Organic Gomasio
**Oindo Umeboshi Plum Paste
**Mitoku's Brown Rice Mochi and Mugwort Mochi
**Sushi Sonic's Organic Toasted Sesame Oil
**San-J's Organic Shoyu
**Ohsawa Organic Kukicha Twig Tea
**Large Variety of Organic Beans, Lentils and Whole Grains
  (Millet, Amaranth, Quinoa)

At Peoples Pharmacy:
**Tonic Alchemy—Greens, Enzymes, Sea Vegetable Drink
**Quantum Probiotic Complex from Premier Research Labs
**Max Stress B Nano-Plex from Premier Research Labs
**Himalayan Crystal Table Salt

Canned Tuna:
Oregon's Choice Gourmet for low mercury tuna: http://www.

oregonschoice.com/ or 541-765-2193. Pacific Northwest Tuna,
it is said to naturally lower in mercury.

Home Delivered Organic Vegetables:
Greenling   at   www.AustinOrganicDelivery.com   or
1.888.789.2352.

Farmers Markets with local Organic produce and Aster's
Ethiopian Food:
Austin Farmers' Market
Sunset Valley Farmers Market

The Heritage Store: 800-862-2923
The Heritage Store offers a large, interesting, natural product
line including Dr Pagano's Recommended Teas for Psoriasis:
Slippery Elm Bark, American Saffron.

The Dirty Dozen are the 12 most contaminated and tainted
Non-Organic foods, i.e. it's more important to buy organic
when buying this specific type of produce. Notice that many
of them on this list are thin skinned.
Apples
Bell peppers
Celery
Cherries
Imported grapes
Nectarines
Peaches
Pears
Potatoes
Red raspberries
Spinach
Strawberries

The 12 Least Tainted, i.e. it's less important to buy organic when buying this produce. Notice that most are thicker skinned.

Asparagus
Avocados
Bananas
Broccoli
Cauliflower
Sweet corn
Kiwi
Mangos
Onions
Papaya
Pineapples
Sweet peas

Chapter Eight
In My Refrigerator

Cut watermelon pieces
Lundberg Farms' Tamari with Seaweed Brown Rice Cakes
Roasted Nuts and Seeds: Walnuts, Tamari Almonds, Pumpkin, Sunflower, Pine Nuts
Dried Fruit—Raisins (all varieties), Cherries, Bananas, Apricots, Berries
South River Miso
Odwalla's Superfood Juice
Oka's Miso Dressing
Fish Oil Supplements
Martin Brothers Dressings: Tamari Vinaigrette, Balsamic Vinaigrette, Thai Peanut
Sass Dressings: Lemon Song, Sesame Garlic, Bombay Ginger
Mixed Organic Salad Greens
Cereal Varieties—Arrowhead Mills Puffed Grains and Fruit Sweetened Cereals
Pacific Brand Almond Milk
Rice Dream Enriched Brown Rice Beverage
Organic Apple Juice

Produce: Organic Celery, Carrots, Shallots, Onions,
   Chives, Garlic, Beets, Leeks, Turnips, Avocado, Arugula,
   Romaine, Limes, Lemons, Squashes, Green Beans,
   Corn, Rapini, Sugar Snap Peas, Asparagus, Burdock
   Root, Daikon, Kale Varieties, Sweet Potatoes, Yams,
   Fennel.
Sea Vegetables: Organic Nori Rolls, Kombu, Wakame, and
   Dulse Granules
Hummus
Whole Organic Spelt Tortillas
100% Maple Syrup
Silken Tofu
Kalamata Olives and Olive Varieties
Bulk Basil Pesto
Unsweetened Applesauce
Pickles and / or Sauerkraut in Salt Brine
Precut Veggies like Baby Carrots, Broccoli Coleslaw, and
   Chinese Veggie Mix
Organic Shoyu
Miso Mayo
Balsamic Vinegar
Ume vinegar
Organic Sesame Oil
Capers
Flax Seeds
Eden Organic Gomasio
Maille Mustard
Teas

In My Freezer:

Precut Frozen Corn, Lima Beans, Black-eyed Peas, Green
   Peas
Frozen Precut Berry Mix, Blueberries, Mango, Pineapple,
   Cherries
Sea Salt

Organic Coffee
Frozen Tilapia and Frozen White Fish Fillets
Steel Cut Oats
Millet, Amaranth

In My Pantry:

Pinto Beans
Locally produced Honey
Sardines in Lemon Juice and Olive Oil
Black pepper, Sea Salt and Turmeric
Cliff Bars, Odwalla Bars, LaraBars
Organic Olive Oil
Roasted Salted Peanuts
Rice or Corn Crackers
Wheat-free Pastas
Rice Noodles
Organic Dry Popped Popcorn

Chapter Nine
In a Restaurant

There are a growing number of restaurants that make it easy to find lunches and dinners of brown rice, fresh and sautéed vegetables, sea vegetables, vegetable or miso soups, pinto beans and rice, fresh fruit and 100% fruit smoothies, sushi rolls wrapped in nori, gluten-free pastas, grilled fish and grilled fish salads. Below is a list of restaurants in Austin, but the general decision principles can be applied anywhere. This list emphasizes restaurants where you can maintain a diet built around whole grains, vegetables, fruits, beans and lentils. If you don't see these things on the menu, ask if they can be made for you. Sometimes restaurants will serve gluten-free and dairy-free items which aren't listed on their menu. I use the excuse of 'food allergies' to request these things, and many times I've marveled at the effort of staff to meet my dietary restrictions.

Zen Japanese Fast Food
Berryhill Baja Tamales and Tacos—spinach/corn tamales,
    rice, beans
NuAge Café
Whole Foods Market

Casa de Luz

PeiWei Asian Diner

Fire Bowl Cafe

East Side Café

West Lynn Café

Hyde Park Bar & Grill—Veggie Platter, Roasted Carrots

Madras Pavilion, Swad and All Indian Restaurants—Vegan options, lentils, rice

Guero's Mexican Food—Corn tortillas, rice, beans, grilled veggies

Uchi, Benihana and All Japanese Restaurants

Polvo's Mexican Food—Grilled Fish with Black Beans and Rice

Magnolia Café—Love Veggies, Black Bean Entrée, Grilled fish with brown rice

Kerby Lane Café—Black Beans and Brown Rice and Sautéed Veggies

Wild Woods Wheat-free Cafe

Luby's—Baked White Fish, Salads, Veggie side dishes

Veggie Heaven

Galaxy Cafe

Cosmic Café

Souper Salad

Fresh Choice

Juice Joint

Mother's Café and Garden

Mr. Natural

World Beat Café and Ethiopian Restaurants—lentils, rice, beans

Ararat—Persian rice, grilled veggies, hummus, baba ganoush

Alborz—Persian rice, grilled veggies, hummus, baba ganoush

Madame Mam's, Thai Noodle, Thai Passion and all Thai Restaurants

Sunflower and all Vietnamese Restaurants

Java Noodle and all Indonesian Restaurants

Seoul Restaurant and all Korean Restaurants

Din Ho, China Palace & Chinese Restaurants—Rice/Rice Noodles, Sautéed Veggies

Italian Restaurants—Grilled fish & veggies, Corn Polenta, Olives, Rice Risotto

Central Market—Grilled Caesar Salmon Salad and Grilled Salmon Dinner Plate

Wendy's—fresh fruit platter

Chipotle—Burrito Bowl with black beans, rice, guacamole and lemon squeezed on top

Chango's—Grilled Mahi Mahi tacos on corn tortillas with black beans

Freebird—Bird Salad or Tacos with black beans and rice on corn tortillas

Taco Cabana—Rice, Black Beans, Cilantro

Baby Greens

Chapter Ten
Traveling

For Traveling, you can pack:

Brown rice cakes, almond butter, local honey, fresh fruit, fresh fruit spreads, cereal, almond milk, hummus, canned tuna, precut veggie sticks, snack bars, vegetarian sushi (with no perishable meat or fish in it), brown rice and precut veggie mixes, salad dressing of vinegar and oil, seeds (pumpkin, sunflower), nuts (almonds, pistachios, walnuts, pecans), raisins, dried fruits, wheat-free fig bars, Veggie Booty and Tings.

Pack a cooler with:

1) Ice
2) Almond milk—individual portions are best but these might only be available in soy milk. With soy milk, it's harder to find options that don't include cane juice. If you are very serious about healing, get rice or almond milk without cane juice. If you can't get individual portions in that, just keep the rice

or almond milk in the cooler with ice. If you use individual portions, you don't have to keep them refrigerated until they're opened.

3)   Salad dressings

4)   Cooked brown rice in a Tupperware container. Just add precut veggies and dressing to this to make a delicious and quick meal.

5)   Precut, prepackaged vegetables—pack these on top of a cooler so they don't get wet, and take some freezer bags or Tupperware containers to keep the melted ice out. You can dip these in almond butter or hummus and add them to rice dishes or eat them plain.

6)   Prepackaged salad greens—add as many dark, leafy veggies as possible. Make a salad or add them on top of dishes.

7)   Individual portion fruit juices

8)   If you can really keep things cold, you may want to take plain, nonfat yogurt.

9)   Fresh fruit that you prefer to eat cold, like grapes.

If you can't have a cooler, all of this will probably hold a few days in a refrigerated hotel room that's shaded from direct sunlight. Put the products as near to the air conditioner as possible. If you take yogurt, the ones which contain only nonfat milk and cultures seem to survive best.

Dry packing:

1)   Cereal

2)   Canned or vacuum packed Light Tuna

3)   Canned Sardines

4)   Rice or gluten-free crackers

5)   Packaged plain oatmeal

6)   Almonds, sliced or whole, to add to oatmeal and other dishes

7) Seeds and nuts to add to dishes and to eat as snacks
8) Any dried unsulphured, unsweetened fruits.
9) LaraBars, Nectar bars and wheat-free fig bars
10) Individually portioned fruit juices like Odwalla Superfood and fresh fruit
11) Almond butter, 100% fruit spreads and local honey
12) Brown Rice Cakes with Seaweed
13) One plate, fork, spoon, knife and reusable cloth napkin per person.
14) Distilled, spring or mineral water

Chapter Eleven
Adopting this Diet and What to Expect

1) Your stools should change for the better. You should have at least one stool per day. To the extent that you have a plant based diet, they will float and resemble a so-called 'golden banana' in appearance.

2) Over time, you can expect a weird discharge. As the body increases its ability to eliminate accumulated toxins, they will come out through stools and other areas such as skin, lungs and reproductive organs. This might be evidenced by a different and heavier menstruation, rashes or a brownish discharge from the skin, or flu-like symptoms. Discharges are temporary but you'll notice them because they will be unusual.

3) When embarking upon a major lifestyle change, it is imperative to surround yourself with supportive people who will facilitate, rather than complicate, your natural healing. Eliminating alcohol and animal products from one's diet can present challenges of social acceptance from family and

friends. Tell them about your decision to use food for natural healing. Ask for their help and give them specific suggestions on how they can support you and increase your chances of success. For example, suggest specific restaurants, let friends know you'll bring a dish to dinner parties that everybody can try, perhaps even ask them to refrain from eating things in front of you that present the biggest temptation.

4) In physical and emotional ways, food and dietary habits are like addictions. Understanding and accepting this before you embark upon diet change will make it easier to move past the anger, withdrawal and feelings of deprivation when they arise. Utilize affirmative statements to counteract these negative feelings. Try to focus on the good your body offers you and be grateful for that, rather than focusing on the illness and dietary restrictions you might be facing.

5) Be prepared to get hungry. My worst choices happen when I'm hungry and unprepared for it. Always keep healthy foods at your fingertips and in your car, purse, home and office to avoid instances when hunger hits and it's impossible to go to the grocery store. LaraBars, Cliff Bars, Roasted Peanuts, Brown Rice Cakes and Almond Butter, Almonds and Raisins, and fruit smoothies all work for me.

6) To give natural healing with food a chance to succeed, I believe it's important to have a very high level of commitment to it for at least six months. Attempt to rarely deviate during that timeframe. After six months and after you've experienced symptom improvement, allow yourself more flexibility. For instance, I was extremely compliant and never ate nightshades for the first six months. Now I have nightshades about once a week. I also eat beef and chicken about 4 times per year, and I drink wine

about 3 times per year. For long-term success with this diet, I believe it helps to do the diet imperfectly. This will allow you to practice a healing diet longer, and it will also ensure that you get a wide variety of nutrients in your diet. I guard one or two cherished foods, like coffee in the morning, to trick my brain from feelings of deprivation and to make it easier to accept practicing this diet for the rest of my life.

Chapter Twelve
Easy, Recipe-Free Meals and Snacks

Breakfast:

1) Whole Grain Cereals. Read ingredient labels to avoid cane juice. Arrowhead Mills and Nature's Path make varieties that are unsweetened or sweetened with fruit juice. Arrowhead Mills makes Puffed Whole Corn, Puffed Whole Millet, Puffed Brown Rice and fruit sweetened Spelt Flakes and Amaranth Flakes. Nature's Path makes fruit sweetened Cornflakes.

2) Sliced Fresh Fruit

3) Steel Cut Oats—with or without raisins, pumpkin seeds, sunflower seeds, sliced fruit, diced dried fruits like apricots, cherries, cranberries. Including a good protein source like seeds or nuts in the cereal will sustain you for a longer period of time before hunger hits again. Steel cut oats are especially recommended for those with heart disease and elevated cholesterol levels.

4) Breakfast Bar like a LaraBar or Nectar bar made

of only nuts and seeds and dried fruit. Avoid all cane juice and processed items in the many options of breakfast and snack bars. Wheat-free, fruit sweetened fig bars.

5) Rice or Almond Milk—Always look for the labels which do not include any cane juice. These beverages are presented as alternatives to dairy milk because many people have allergies to dairy. Dairy is mucus-forming, meaning that it slows down the elimination process versus facilitating it, and hence cow's dairy should be avoided as much as possible.

6) Odwalla's Super Food or B-Monster Fruit Juices. Naked Juices. Sambazon's Organic Acai Energy Drinks without cane juice. Amazake Brown Rice Drinks without cane juice.

7) Breakfast at one of the listed restaurants.

Recipe-free, fast Lunches and Dinners:

1) Cooked brown rice is always in my refrigerator. Put Precut Vegetables (Chinese Veggie Mix, Coleslaw, Broccoli Slaw, etc) atop brown rice (or any cooked whole grain). Add variety by alternating various precut veggies and salad dressings. Oka's Miso Dressing is my favorite. I love the flavor and the second ingredient is miso. Martin Brothers and SASS dressings use apple cider vinegar and fresh ingredients, so I buy them frequently.

2) Take the same dish above except add your own vegetables with or without more precut vegetables. I often cook brown rice with turnips and sweet potato and yams. To make the rice, I use 2 parts water to 1 part brown rice with sea salt and an ice-cube sized chunk of kombu. Bring the rice and water to a boil, turn the temperature down very low to maintain a slow boil, put the lid on the pot and set the timer

for 35 minutes. The rice is done when there's no standing water in the bottom of the pot. When the rice has finished cooking, I turn off the heat, remove the kombu and top the steaming brown rice with chopped vegetables of any kind except nightshades. Then I put the lid back on to cover everything in the pot so that the steam from the rice will lightly cook the rest of the vegetables. My favorite vegetables for this dish are asparagus, fresh cut corn from the husk, carrots, burdock root, daikon radish, celery, bok choy, green cabbage, beets, kale, beets, turnips, collard greens, arugula and scallions. I always put the dark leafy greens at the top of the pot so that they steam the least. Serve on a bed of mixed salad greens or arugula, sprinkle with dulse granules and gomasio, and then top it with your favorite dressing.

3) Hummus wrapped in a whole spelt tortilla with kalamata olives, mixed greens and arugula.

4) Miso Soup with wakame.

5) Tuna Salad made with Miso Mayo, and any mixture of many vegetables. I mix in broccoli slaw, coleslaw, carrots, grapes, seeds, celery, fresh cut corn and turmeric. Then I wrap this tuna salad in a whole spelt tortilla.

6) Brown rice cakes with seaweed, almond butter and 100% fruit spread, fresh fruit, dried fruit or honey.

7) Lundberg Farm brown rice cakes with tamari and seaweed, Tohum brand roasted tahini, 100% fruit spread or fresh fruit or honey.

8) For a quick soup, you can use any fresh or frozen vegetable except nightshades. Place in a pot, cover the veggies with water, add sliced onions and celery and sea salt and pepper, bring to a boil and cook until done. Puree the cooked vegetables for a delicious

pureed soup. Garnish with cilantro, scallions or parsley.

9) Sardines in Olive Oil with Rice crackers.

10) Fresh veggie plate with hummus or pesto and olives.

11) Aster's Ethiopian Teff bread with mild lentils and spinach side dishes.

12) Steel cut oats with sunflower seeds or sliced almonds, dried or fresh fruit, flax seeds.

13) Recommended cereal with banana and almond milk.

14) Fruit smoothie with nonfat, organic, plain yogurt, frozen fruit of choice and organic apple juice.

15) Precut fruit and vegetables and organic goat cheese with fresh squeezed lemon juice.

16) Steamed white fish with any assortment of vegetables on a bed of mixed greens.

17) Any of the restaurants provided.

Snack Foods

1) Lundberg Farms Whole Grain Rice Cakes— Tamari with Seaweed is the best choice. They also make fabulous brown rice chips with sesame and seaweed.

2) Almond Butter with 100% fruit spreads on a brown rice cake. 100% fruit is recommended over honey, but honey is a much better choice than a white sugar alternative. You can also add whole fruit, raisins, etc.

3) Any nut butter which includes just the nuts and sea salt (i.e. the fewest ingredients possible). Almonds are the best nut because they are the only nut which yields alkalinity.

4) Breads with fewer ingredients. Food for Life's Spelt

Bread and Sprouted Grain breads. Whole organic spelt tortillas.

5) Veggie Booty by Robert's American Gourmet (Puffed Rice and Corn with Spinach and Kale) and their other veggie snacks. This same company makes delicious "Tings" and "Fruity Booty".

6) Barbara's Natural Choice Granola Bars which are sweetened with Honey and contain no cane sweeteners. LaraBars and Nectar Bars. Odwalla Bars without cane juice.

7) Roasted peanuts in the shell. Tamari roasted almonds and raw or roasted seeds.

8) Date Coconut bars at Whole Foods Market.

9) Steamed Edamame with sea salt.

10) Wheat-free, fruit juice sweetened, raspberry fig bars.

11) Garden of Eden chips and other brands (like Fritos) with a short ingredient list including only corn, corn oil, sea salt. Organic, dry popped popcorn with sea salt.

12) Toasted tamari almonds and raisins.

13) Nori sheets dipped in hummus and homemade sushi with your choice of vegetables and sauces. Sushi is relatively easy to make and would be a fun project for kids.

14) Arrowhead Mills whole grain cereals. There are puffed and fruit sweetened options including Multigrain Flakes, Amaranth Flakes, Spelt Flakes, Kamut Flakes, Puffed Organic Millet, Puffed Corn, Puffed Kamut and Puffed Brown Rice.

15) Vegetable soup with any vegetables. Chop the vegetables, add them to the pot and cover them with water. It's better to add too little water than too much of it because you can always add more water later. Add sea salt, celery, onions, and garlic. Bring to a boil, cover the pot and simmer on low heat until

all vegetables are at your preferred texture. Puree as desired. You can also use frozen vegetables like peas and corn to avoid chopping vegetables. Pasta or rice noodles can be added and it's best to boil the vegetables separately from the noodles. Hard squashes and root vegetables like potatoes and sweet potatoes take longer to cook, so you'll want to throw them in the pot at the beginning. Add miso when desired but be sure to add it AFTER the water has stopped boiling to avoid killing the good bacteria ("probiotics") in it. If you're not accustomed to miso flavor, white miso is sweet and an easier introduction to the flavor of miso than the heavier barley miso. However, the older barley miso offers the best healing benefits.

16) Odwalla Juices especially Super Food and B Monster. Naked Juice, Sambazon and Amazake brand beverages offer lots of flavors without cane juice.

17) Sardines in olive oil on rice crackers.

18) Unsweetened, organic applesauce and apples.

This book is written for Pop because I promised him that someday I'd write a book.

Thank you for sharing your time and please let me know how I can help you to experience the incredible healing power of food!

Deirdre Earls, RD, LD

www.YourHealingDiet.com

(512) 453-8784

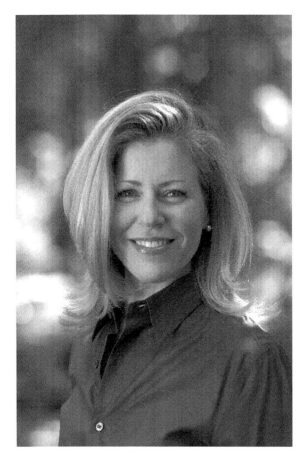

About Deirdre Earls, RD, LD

Deirdre Earls, RD, LD, graduated with honors in Scientific Nutrition from Texas A&M University and her healthcare career spans over 20 years. Having reversed her own severe psoriasis with nutrition instead of chemotherapy drugs, she has been published in Prevention Magazine and is a featured speaker for internationally recognized organizations such as Whole Foods Market and The National Psoriasis Foundation. Ms. Earls' nutrition practice provides personalized dietary guidance that emphasizes natural healing with food for those with busy lifestyles. Her new guidebook, "Your Healing Diet", was written to make it easier than ever before to experience the healing power of food. For more information, please visit her website at www.YourHealingDiet.com or call (512) 453-8784.

Made in the USA
Lexington, KY
20 June 2012